CANCER

CANCER

Biblical
TRUTHS
— *that* —
Bring
Comfort

B&H
PUBLISHING GROUP
NASHVILLE, TENNESSEE

978-1-5359-1770-4

Published by B&H Publishing Group
Nashville, Tennessee

Dewey Decimal Classification: 242.5
Subject Heading: DEVOTIONAL LITERATURE \
BIBLE—INSPIRATION \ MEDITATIONS \ PRAYERS

1 2 3 4 5 6 7 8 • 22 21 20 19 18

CONTENTS

CONTENTS

It's terrible. You went in for a screening. It was only supposed to be a check up. You were supposed to go in, be told that there's something you need to improve, and leave, but that didn't happen. Instead, you're being told that there's something that needs to be taken care of immediately. You're being told that it's going to be a long road. You're being told that there are treatments available. This is a terrible account of how most cancer stories start.

Hundreds of thousands of people receive this diagnosis each year. There are over a million new cases expected to be diagnosed each year. Whether you are the recipient of this news or the family of the recipient, it's a difficult reality to come to terms with. How do we handle this dark time in life? We have to accept it; we have to move past the anger and respond in faithfulness. We have to move forward. We have to deal with the stress and fear that is almost guaranteed to come, and trust that God will protect us.

It is one of the hardest paths some will ever have to walk. It is lonely, fearful, and full of anxiety, but it is also a time where God shines. Families come together; people learn to rely on Him again. Faith is tested and restored. It is a time that most mark as a time of great hardship, but on the other end is rest in God.

Acceptance is the last stage of grief. It is the most difficult of the stages for people to reach. Accepting something does not signify one's giving up, but it does address that there is a problem, and you're ready to deal with it. Cancer is one of the biggest problems you may ever face, but know that you are loved by a God that accepts you and loves you and will walk with you through this time. When we accept this, then we can start moving forward with Him.

But the LORD *said to Samuel, "Do not look at his appearance or his stature because I have rejected him. Humans do not see what the* LORD *sees, for humans see what is visible, but the* LORD *sees the heart."*

    1 Samuel 16:7

———

"Everyone the Father gives me will come to me, and the one who comes to me I will never cast out."

    John 6:37

———

But God proves his own love for us in that while we were still sinners, Christ died for us.

    Romans 5:8

If God is for us, who is against us?
    Romans 8:31

———

Peter began to speak: "Now I truly understand that God doesn't show favoritism, but in every nation the person who fears him and does what is right is acceptable to him.
    Acts 10:34–35

Heavenly Father, I am uncertain of the path that is before me. I don't know what obstacles will be along the road. I am nervous. I feel that I won't be able to handle any of the things that will come from this, but I accept that I am on this path. Lord, walk with me during this time. Allow me to come out of this path with peace in knowing that You are with me. Amen

Anger is a common response to the news of cancer. When one woman received her diagnosis, she smiled and said that there must be some sort of mistake. Not five minutes later she shoved a table and screamed, "NO!" During this time, the doctor simply observed and stayed calm. When asked about how he kept his cool, he simply noted, "It's common for patients to lash out at the news, but as long as they are willing to calm down and talk about how to handle it, then we will move forward." Anger is a reaction, don't let it turn to wrath and fester. Instead, stand with God, and take on that which is before you.

Refrain from anger and give up your rage;
do not be agitated—it can only bring harm.
    Psalm 37:8

———

A patient person shows great understanding,
but a quick-tempered one promotes foolishness.
    Proverbs 14:29

———

A gentle answer turns away anger,
but a harsh word stirs up wrath.
    Proverbs 15:1

"But I tell you, everyone who is angry with his brother or sister will be subject to judgment. Whoever insults his brother or sister, will be subject to the court. Whoever says, 'You fool!' will be subject to hellfire."

Matthew 5:22

———

Be angry and do not sin. Don't let the sun go down on your anger, and don't give the devil an opportunity.

Ephesians 4:26–27

Lord, I am angry. I feel like this is so unfair. I'm upset that I have this burden placed on me. Lord, I know I cannot stay here. I know that I cannot allow this anger to build. I know I need to let it go and move forward with You. Lord, calm my spirit. Allow me to listen to what needs to be said. Father, be with me, and remind me that if I stay angry, healing will only be more difficult. Amen

Few people take the time to realize the kind of anxiety a person experiences during treatment. Chemotherapy and radiation therapy are the two most common forms of treatment. Patients typically hate these treatment sessions because of the side effects that are almost guaranteed by them. Pain, nausea, and fatigue are the most common. Though many patients are anxious about the possibility of death, they are almost just as anxious over the road to recovery. Know that God is with you during this anxious time, and that with Him, you will get through this!

"Therefore I tell you: Don't worry about your life, what you will eat or what you will drink; or about your body, what you will wear. Isn't life more than food and the body more than clothing? Consider the birds of the sky: They don't sow or reap or gather into barns, yet your heavenly Father feeds them. Aren't you worth more than they? Can any of you add one moment to his life-span by worrying?"

Matthew 6:25–27

———

Humble yourselves, therefore, under the mighty hand of God, so that he may exalt you at the proper time, casting all your cares on him, because he cares about you.

1 Peter 5:6–7

"Peace I leave with you. My peace I give to you. I do not give to you as the world gives. Don't let your heart be troubled or fearful."

John 14:27

———

Don't worry about anything, but in everything, through prayer and petition with thanksgiving, present your requests to God. And the peace of God, which surpasses all understanding, will guard your hearts and minds in Christ Jesus.

Philippians 4:6–7

———

For God has not given us a spirit of fear, but one of power, love, and sound judgment.

2 Timothy 1:7

Heavenly Father, I am nervous about the road before me. I am anxious about the unknown. Please allow me to give my anxiety to You. Allow me, Father, to be able to let go of this anxiety and take hold of You. I know that there are going to moments where I stumble. Lord, don't let these moments hold me down. Allow me to stand and move forward with You. Amen

A young girl battled leukemia at the age of fifteen. She had long beautiful blonde hair, but as the treatments started, her hair started to thin and eventually fell out. She was devastated for a few weeks. She wore head scarves every Wednesday and Sunday at church. One Sunday she had had enough. She shaved the rest of her head and walked brazenly down the aisle of the church and took her seat. Years later, when she recounts the story, she remarks that it was the most beautiful she had ever felt since the day she received her diagnosis. Walking with confidence is often the most necessary thing to feeling beautiful. Walk with God and find that beauty.

*I have asked one thing from the L*ORD*;*
it is what I desire:
*to dwell in the house of the L*ORD
all the days of my life,
*gazing on the beauty of the L*ORD
and seeking him in his temple.
   Psalm 27:4

———

I will praise you
because I have been remarkably and wondrously
made.
Your works are wondrous,
and I know this very well.
   Psalm 139:14

Charm is deceptive and beauty is fleeting,
but a woman who fears the LORD will be praised.
  Proverbs 31:30

———

You are absolutely beautiful, my darling;
there is no imperfection in you.
  Song of Songs 4:7

———

Don't let your beauty consist of outward things like
elaborate hairstyles and wearing gold jewelry, but
rather what is inside the heart—the imperishable
quality of a gentle and quiet spirit, which is of great
worth in God's sight.
  1 Peter 3:3–4

Lord, I feel like there is no beauty in this time. I feel sick all of the time. I feel weak. I feel a great amount of things, but none of them make me feel beautiful. Father, I know that this beauty is found in You. Allow me to walk through this process confidently and take hold of You. Allow me to rely on Your leadership in my life and find beauty in the moments that You provide. Amen

There's a family among cancer patients. You get synched up with another patient and your therapies are typically on the same days. Strangers in waiting rooms become acquaintances, then to friendships, to close friendships, and then to family. It is one of the blessings most cancer patients refer to in that they are able to know that they didn't walk that path alone. Some will even remark that God put those people in their lives so that they would not walk alone.

"May the LORD bless you and protect you; may the LORD make his face shine on you and be gracious to you; may the LORD look with favor on you and give you peace."

Numbers 6:24–26

Indeed, we have all received grace upon grace from his fullness, for the law was given through Moses; grace and truth came through Jesus Christ.

John 1:16–17

And God is able to make every grace overflow to you, so that in every way, always having everything you need, you may excel in every good work.

    2 Corinthians 9:8

———

Blessed is the God and Father of our Lord Jesus Christ, who has blessed us with every spiritual blessing in the heavens in Christ.

    Ephesians 1:3

———

And my God will supply all your needs according to his riches in glory in Christ Jesus.

    Philippians 4:19

Father, thank You for the blessings in life. I know that there are times that I choose to focus on the negativity of this time, but during it, You have provided laughter, joy, friendships, and other positives that I've let be overshadowed by the negative. Allow me to focus on the blessings You've provided, Lord. Allow me to count them day by day. Amen

Care is one of the most important parts of the healing process. Many spouses will talk about the moments in which they had to care for their other halves while they were in treatment. Some of their stories would be enough to bring tears to your eyes, but what people always seem to notice about the narrator's story is that there's rarely a tear, but often a joy. If you ask them why, they'll tell you that it's hard to watch someone you love suffer, but it's easy and a joy to care for them during that time of suffering.

"I give you a new command: Love one another. Just as I have loved you, you are also to love one another. By this everyone will know that you are my disciples, if you love one another."
     John 13:34–35

———

Carry one another's burdens; in this way you will fulfill the law of Christ.
     Galatians 6:2

Therefore, as we have opportunity, let us work for the good of all, especially for those who belong to the household of faith.

Galatians 6:10

———

Everyone should look out not only for his own interests, but also for the interests of others.

Philippians 2:4

Heavenly Father, thank You for putting those special people in my life that care for me. I know that I am not easy to care for, and still, You provide those that love me enough to care for me in my time of need. Remind me to repay the kindness others have shown me by caring for others. Amen

It's difficult to understand how we can be a child of God and yet thrown into such suffering. It's something that a lot of people struggle with when they discuss the hardships of dealing with cancer. Like a child, we blame God for the hardships in our lives, but we so often forget that God loves us, and that it is with that love that you will make it through this. You will find peace if you are walking with God. If not, like an unforgiving child, you will only be angry with Him.

"Blessed are the peacemakers, for they will be called sons of God."

>   *Matthew 5:9*

But to all who did receive him, he gave them the right to be children of God, to those who believe in his name, who were born, not of natural descent, or of the will of the flesh, or of the will of man, but of God.

>   *John 1:12–13*

For through faith you are all sons of God in Christ Jesus.

>   *Galatians 3:26*

The Spirit himself testifies together with our spirit that we are God's children, and if children, also heirs—heirs of God and coheirs with Christ—if indeed we suffer with him so that we may also be glorified with him.

Romans 8:16–17

———

See what great love the Father has given us that we should be called God's children—and we are! The reason the world does not know us is that it didn't know him.

1 John 3:1

Father, I am hurting. I am tired, and I am desperate for You. Father, I am so sorry for my anger when I've directed it toward You. I know that was wrong. I know that You love me, and I'm sorry that I turned from You in my frustrations. Lord, allow me to walk with You. Remind me of Your love daily. Thank You for loving me, Lord. Amen

One mother talks about the pain and heartache that came from her treatments and how most days were a struggle just to get out of bed, but when she was asked about what brought her comfort, she talked about her faith and her young son. She said that whenever she was having a bad day, he would simply sit next to the bed and hold her hand while they watched a movie together. We have no idea the level of comfort we bring to someone if we just sit with them and love them. Seek God and find comfort in the times of pain.

Even when I go through the darkest valley,
I fear no danger,
for you are with me;
your rod and your staff—they comfort me.
   Psalm 23:4

———

Remember your word to your servant;
you have given me hope through it.
This is my comfort in my affliction:
Your promise has given me life.
   Psalm 119:49–50

———

As a mother comforts her son, so I will comfort you,
and you will be comforted in Jerusalem.
   Isaiah 66:13

"Blessed are those who mourn, for they will be comforted."

Matthew 5:4

———

Blessed be the God and Father of our Lord Jesus Christ, the Father of mercies and the God of all comfort. He comforts us in all our affliction, so that we may be able to comfort those who are in any kind of affliction, through the comfort we ourselves receive from God.

2 Corinthians 1:3–4

Lord, I am in need of Your comfort. I feel like the pain and fatigue in my life is overwhelming and I can no longer live like this. I need peace, Lord. I need comfort. Father, calm my uneasiness and allow me to find comfort in You. Amen

CONFIDENCE

Confidence is a rare commodity in most cancer patients. Most of the time the news is so devastating that it takes almost all of their willpower not to break down and cry right there, but every once in awhile, you find that rarity. When Jacob was told that his chances were slim, he grinned and said sarcastically "It wouldn't be fun if it were easy . . ." He put his mind to the test. He exercised every day. Even on days that he could barely move, he got up and walked at the very least. After months of therapy, his health started to turn around, he began to recover. Today, he still has screenings every six months, but stands by words he would say to his doctor at every appointment. "Just because it's hard doesn't make it impossible."

Do not fear, for I am with you; do not be afraid, for I am your God. I will strengthen you; I will help you; I will hold on to you with my righteous right hand.
  Isaiah 41:10

———

It is not that we are competent in ourselves to claim anything as coming from ourselves, but our adequacy is from God.
  2 Corinthians 3:5

———

I am able to do all things through him who strengthens me.
  Philippians 4:13

So don't throw away your confidence, which has a great reward. For you need endurance, so that after you have done God's will, you may receive what was promised.

   Hebrews 10:35–36

This is how we will know that we belong to the truth and will reassure our hearts before him whenever our hearts condemn us; for God is greater than our hearts, and he knows all things. Dear friends, if our hearts don't condemn us, we have confidence before God and receive whatever we ask from him because we keep his commands and do what is pleasing in his sight.

   1 John 3:19–22

Father, I don't feel ready to take on this obstacle. I feel that I am going to fail during this time in my life. Every day I feel like I won't be strong enough to succeed. Father, take this spirit away from me and instill in me a confidence that knows I will succeed. Allow me to wake up and just know that whatever may come before me, You are with me. Amen

Finding contentment seems impossible with cancer. One woman's journey tested that notion. She was a leader at her company, and when she received the diagnosis, she realized very quickly that she was going to have to give that up. She had put years into the company and then it was gone. The company said they would simply find an interim, but she knew she was going to be gone for at least a year. She was restless for the first few months of her treatment. Something changed when she developed a friendship with a department store manager. He looked at her and said, "The treatment is rough, but at least I don't have to do inventory . . ." After he said that, she realized that she was getting rest from meetings, spreadsheets, and business lunches. For once, she was able to focus on herself. The treatment was difficult, but she was able to let go of the responsibilities of work and take on the responsibilities of her life.

*"So don't worry, saying, 'What will we eat?' or
'What will we drink?' or 'What will we wear?'
For the Gentiles eagerly seek all these things,
and your heavenly Father knows that you need
them. But seek first the kingdom of God and his
righteousness, and all these things will be provided
for you. Therefore don't worry about tomorrow,
because tomorrow will worry about itself. Each day
has enough trouble of its own."*

Matthew 6:31–34

———

*But godliness with contentment is great gain. For
we brought nothing into the world, and we can take
nothing out. If we have food and clothing, we will
be content with these.*

1 Timothy 6:6–8

He then told them, "Watch out and be on guard against all greed, because one's life is not in the abundance of his possessions."
   Luke 12:15

———

I don't say this out of need, for I have learned to be content in whatever circumstances I find myself. I know both how to make do with little, and I know how to make do with a lot. In any and all circumstances I have learned the secret of being content—whether well fed or hungry, whether in abundance or in need.
   Philippians 4:11–12

Heavenly Father, I feel like there is nothing I can be content about during this time. I feel that no matter what I do I cannot recognize the things that would give me contentment. Lord, remind me to find my contentment in You. Allow me to know that there are things that You have given me that will produce a content heart. Allow me to recognize those things, Lord. Amen

Courage does not equal fearlessness. It is something that most of us know and yet choose to ignore whenever we hear or read the word. Treatment is one of those things that requires a great deal of courage. People hate to come to terms with the fact that they're scared after receiving the diagnosis, but they still have to move forward. Take courage in knowing that the hard times will pass, and you can courageously walk forward with God.

"Haven't I commanded you: be strong and courageous? Do not be afraid or discouraged, for the LORD your God is with you wherever you go."
    Joshua 1:9

———

I always let the LORD guide me.
Because he is at my right hand,
I will not be shaken.
    Psalm 16:8

Wait for the LORD*;*
be strong, and let your heart be courageous.
Wait for the LORD*.*
>   *Psalm 27:14*

———

Be alert, stand firm in the faith, be courageous, be
strong.
>   *1 Corinthians 16:13*

———

For God has not given us a spirit of fear, but one of
power, love, and sound judgment.
>   *2 Timothy 1:7*

Lord, I feel like I won't be able to overcome this. I know that I cannot do it on my own, and for that, I am scared. Lord, take away this fearful spirit and allow me to move forward in courage with You. Amen

Most cancer patients often deal with depression at least once on their path to recovery. During this time, depression is debilitating. It's a pool you can sink into and never seem to reach the bottom; it just feels like you go deeper and deeper. Depression, however, is not a place to stay. Depression is a place for the defeated, and that is something we are not called to ever be. Take hold of Christ and climb out of this depression and claim victory with Him.

The LORD sits enthroned over the flood;
the LORD sits enthroned, King forever.
The LORD gives his people strength;
the LORD blesses his people with peace.
  Psalm 29:10–11

———

The LORD is near the brokenhearted;
he saves those crushed in spirit.
  Psalm 34:18

———

I will give you the treasures of darkness and riches
from secret places, so that you may know that I am
the LORD. I am the God of Israel, who calls you by
your name.
  Isaiah 45:3

Answer me quickly, LORD;
my spirit fails.
Don't hide your face from me,
or I will be like those
going down to the Pit.
Let me experience
your faithful love in the morning,
for I trust in you.
Reveal to me the way I should go
because I appeal to you.
    Psalm 143:7–8

———

Do not fear, for I am with you; do not be afraid, for I
am your God. I will strengthen you; I will help you;
I will hold on to you with my righteous right hand.
    Isaiah 41:10

Lord Jesus, I am crushed. I am beaten down, and I don't know how I can go on. I know that through You there is victory. Lord, allow me to chase after You daily so that I may find that victory. Allow me to climb out of this depression by taking hold of You. Amen

When you first get the news of your diagnosis, it's a discouraging feeling. That goes without saying. It's a reaction to bad news of any kind, but this is a very specific kind of discouragement. This is a feeling of defeat before the battle has even started. It's a reaction most patients acknowledge within the first five minutes of the diagnosis. A discouragement, however, is merely a setback. Cancer may be the biggest setback we could ever get, but are we letting this discouragement operate more like a defeat? Take hold of God and move forward, past the discouragement and onward with Him.

The LORD is the one who will go before you. He will be with you; he will not leave you or abandon you. Do not be afraid or discouraged.

   Deuteronomy 31:8

———

"I have told you these things so that in me you may have peace. You will have suffering in this world. Be courageous! I have conquered the world."

   John 16:33

———

Now may the God of hope fill you with all joy and peace as you believe so that you may overflow with hope by the power of the Holy Spirit.

   Romans 15:13

In the same way the Spirit also helps us in our weakness, because we do not know what to pray for as we should, but the Spirit himself intercedes for us with unspoken groanings. And he who searches our hearts knows the mind of the Spirit, because he intercedes for the saints according to the will of God. We know that all things work together for the good of those who love God, who are called according to his purpose.

    Romans 8:26–28

———

But he said to me, "My grace is sufficient for you, for my power is perfected in weakness."
Therefore, I will most gladly boast all the more about my weaknesses, so that Christ's power may reside in me.

    2 Corinthians 12:9

Father, I am devastated. I am crushed. I feel like I won't be able to overcome what is in front of me. Lord, I know that I cannot do this on my own. I know that it is not through my will, alone, that I will be able to take on the obstacles before me. Lord, be with me. Walk with me as I take on the walls that stand before me. Amen

One of the things you'll often hear from patients is a sense of dissatisfaction. They are often impatient during their care. One patient once yelled at his doctor, "With these side effects, I should be healing faster!" After a month of his complaints, the doctor finally sat him down with a chart showing his cancer cells. He showed how they looked at the diagnosis and how they looked four months later. They had shrunk, not considerably, but shrinking all the same. The doctor finally said, "The fact that they're shrinking at all is something that should bring you a little peace. It's when they stop shrinking that we find a problem." How many times have we been impatient because we expect God to move the way we want Him to move?

For he has satisfied the thirsty
and filled the hungry with good things.
  Psalm 107:9

———

You open your hand
and satisfy the desire of every living thing.
  Psalm 145:16

———

The LORD will always lead you, satisfy you in a
parched land, and strengthen your bones.
You will be like a watered garden and like a spring
whose water never runs dry.
  Isaiah 58:11

"I am the bread of life," Jesus told them. "No one who comes to me will ever be hungry, and no one who believes in me will ever be thirsty again."

John 6:35

———

Now may the God of hope fill you with all joy and peace as you believe so that you may overflow with hope by the power of the Holy Spirit.

Romans 15:13

Heavenly Father, I know that I have been impatient. I know that I have been dissatisfied lately. I don't want to wait for anything any longer. I know that I need to learn the importance of being patient and satisfied with what is currently before me. Lord, instill in me a spirit of patience and satisfaction so that I may be able to be thankful for what I have presently and be hopeful for whatever may come. Amen

There was a patient being treated with chemotherapy. Her body was weak; she was tired, but with everything she had, she walked with confidence. Once a month she would walk in for treatment and yell at the waiting room, "One Cycle Down!" The people would laugh and clap as she walked into the doctor's office. After her therapy was finished, she stayed nearby, and every time a person would walk in that door for the start of a new cycle she would make sure to whisper that they were one cycle closer to being finished. An encouraging word, even just a sentence, can bring strength to those that are being brought into weakening situations.

*The LORD is the one who will go before you. He will
be with you; he will not leave you or abandon you.
Do not be afraid or discouraged.*

   Deuteronomy 31:8

———

*God is our refuge and strength,
a helper who is always found in times of trouble.*

   Psalm 46:1

———

*"Aren't five sparrows sold for two pennies? Yet not
one of them is forgotten in God's sight. Indeed, the
hairs of your head are all counted. Don't be afraid;
you are worth more than many sparrows."*

   Luke 12:6–7

"I have told you these things so that in me you may have peace. You will have suffering in this world. Be courageous! I have conquered the world."
   John 16:33

———

And let us watch out for one another to provoke love and good works, not neglecting to gather together, as some are in the habit of doing, but encouraging each other, and all the more as you see the day approaching.
   Hebrews 10:24–25

Lord, thank You for those that give encouraging words as I go through hard times. Allow that encouragement to continue in my life. Father, remind me to take the encouragement that has been given to me and share that with those that need it as well. Allow me to be gracious when people cheer for me, and allow me to encourage when I cheer for others. Amen

One of the lessons that young cancer patients will tell you they've learned is the heavy lesson of their own mortality. They learn that nothing lasts forever, and that life on this world is temporary. It's not uncommon that you hear patients discover Christ while in treatment. One of the things one patient discusses in his story is this, "When you're reminded of how temporary everything in this world is, it seems almost natural to focus what is eternal."

Before the mountains were born,
before you gave birth to the earth and the world,
from eternity to eternity, you are God.

    Psalm 90:2

———

He has made everything appropriate in its time.
He has also put eternity in their hearts, but no
one can discover the work God has done from
beginning to end.

    Ecclesiastes 3:11

———

"This is eternal life: that they may know you, the
only true God, and the one you have sent—Jesus
Christ."

    John 17:3

"Truly I tell you, anyone who hears my word and believes him who sent me has eternal life and will not come under judgment but has passed from death to life."

    John 5:24

———

For the wages of sin is death, but the gift of God is eternal life in Christ Jesus our Lord.

    Romans 6:23

*Father, it seems that nothing lasts forever.
In this world, nothing is eternal. Lord, everything
seems to have an expiration date . . . everything
except You. Father, thank You for being there.
Thank You for having a love for me that
always has been and always will be. Amen*

Living a faithful life in an uneasy time is one of the hardest things to do. It's especially difficult when trying to move forward after a cancer diagnosis. One woman in particular had an interesting story on her faith. She read the Bible during her chemotherapy sessions to pass the time. When another patient would ask her why she wasted her time reading "that book." Her response was simple, "My medicine, my doctor, and my health may fail, but God will never fail me . . . no matter what happens. I have a God that loves me and is preparing a place for me. Am I ready to go home? I don't know . . . but I know that I have a home to go to."

Because of the LORD*'s faithful love we do not perish,*
for his mercies never end. They are new every
morning; great is your faithfulness!
    Lamentations 3:22–23

"His master said to him, 'Well done, good and
faithful servant! You were faithful over a few
things; I will put you in charge of many things.
Share your master's joy.'"
    Matthew 25:21

If we are faithless, he remains faithful, for he
cannot deny himself.
    2 Timothy 2:13

"Whoever is faithful in very little is also faithful in much, and whoever is unrighteous in very little is also unrighteous in much. So if you have not been faithful with worldly wealth, who will trust you with what is genuine? And if you have not been faithful with what belongs to someone else, who will give you what is your own?"
    Luke 16:10–12

———

Let us hold on to the confession of our hope without wavering, since he who promised is faithful.
    Hebrews 10:23

Lord Jesus, thank You for preparing a place for me. Thank You for dying for my sins. During the hard times, allow me to maintain my focus on You. Instill in me a spirit that lives out a life of faithfulness. Lord, remind me daily of Your love, grace, and mercy, and allow me to respond in faith. Amen

After the diagnosis, fear is one of the most natural responses that we find in patients. It is a reaction to the unknown, but to let it linger is something that will evolve to fear if you allow it. Cancer can seem like one of the most terrifying seasons in your life, but we are not called to live in fear. Take courage and move forward with God.

"Haven't I commanded you: be strong and courageous? Do not be afraid or discouraged, for the LORD *your God is with you wherever you go."*
  Joshua 1:9

———

When I am afraid,
I will trust in you.
  Psalm 56:3

———

You did not receive a spirit of slavery to fall back into fear. Instead, you received the Spirit of adoption, by whom we cry out, "Abba, Father!"
  Romans 8:15

For God has not given us a spirit of fear, but one of power, love, and sound judgment.
    2 Timothy 1:7

————

Humble yourselves, therefore, under the mighty hand of God, so that he may exalt you at the proper time, casting all your cares on him, because he cares about you.
    1 Peter 5:6–7

Heavenly Father, I am afraid. I am afraid of the path that is before me. I don't know what's on it. I don't know what all I will have to do, and that worries me. Lord, I know that with You, I have nothing to fear. Continue to allow me to lean on You, Father. Amen

The future is an uneasy concept to think about when going through therapy. It almost feels like you're not allowed to think about it until after you've been cured. One father had been planning a trip with his family for a couple of months when he was diagnosed. It was going to be a few years away. He didn't stop planning it. When the family was able to go, one of his children asked him why he didn't stop planning. The father's response was, "If I stopped planning, that would've meant that I had given up. I wasn't about to do that." When we have faith that God is with us, then the future does not seem as uneasy.

The L*ORD* *will fulfill his purpose for me.*
L*ORD*, *your faithful love endures forever;*
do not abandon the work of your hands.
    Psalm 138:8

———

A person's heart plans his way,
but the L*ORD* *determines his steps.*
    Proverbs 16:9

———

For I know the plans I have for you"—this is the
L*ORD's declaration—"plans for your well-being, not*
for disaster, to give you a future and a hope.
    Jeremiah 29:11

But our citizenship is in heaven, and we eagerly wait for a Savior from there, the Lord Jesus Christ. He will transform the body of our humble condition into the likeness of his glorious body, by the power that enables him to subject everything to himself.

   Philippians 3:20–21

———

Dear friends, we are God's children now, and what we will be has not yet been revealed. We know that when he appears, we will be like him because we will see him as he is.

   1 John 3:2

Father, I'm so afraid to think about what tomorrow holds. I know that I just need to give it to You. Allow me to do that, Lord. Allow me to give my fears on the future to You. Allow me to be able to focus on the positive of what tomorrow may hold and not live in fear of the negative. Amen

When the doctor told a teenage girl that healing would take a little more time, the mother had had just about enough. She stood to her feet, slapped the clipboard out of the doctor's hand, and yelled, "Are you even trying?!" She stormed out of the room, sure that she was going to have to find another doctor. The doctor, however, waited patiently with her daughter. When the mother returned to apologize, the doctor listened and said, "You're not the first mother that's yelled at me . . . you won't be the last . . . just be patient. We are doing the best that we can." Grace is about recognizing where people are at and moving forward, regardless of how they fall. God does the same for us, God grants us grace, not because we deserve it, but because He loves us.

The law came along to multiply the trespass. But where sin multiplied, grace multiplied even more.
   Romans 5:20

———

For sin will not rule over you, because you are not under the law but under grace.
   Romans 6:14

———

Now if by grace, then it is not by works; otherwise grace ceases to be grace.
   Romans 11:6

But he said to me, "My grace is sufficient for you, for my power is perfected in weakness." Therefore, I will most gladly boast all the more about my weaknesses, so that Christ's power may reside in me.

2 Corinthians 12:9

———

For you are saved by grace through faith, and this is not from yourselves; it is God's gift—not from works, so that no one can boast.

Ephesians 2:8–9

Lord, I'm sorry. I have been impatient, fearful, and angry. I know that's not how You've called us to live. Father, there are so many times in life that I don't deserve Your love and grace, and yet, You still give it to me. Thank You, Father. Thank You for constantly loving me even in my times when I feel unlovable. Amen

Cancer can sometimes bring loss. We know that brings grief as well, but what you do with that grief is up to you. One of the most famous losses to this disease is Walt Disney. With his death, the family was left with a choice, they could either let grief settle and take root in their family, or they could move forward with something bigger. There was a theme park Walt and his brother, Roy, had been planning for quite some time. As a tribute to his brother, Roy named the park and the company after Walt, and with that grief the family chose to stand up and spread as much joy to the world as they could.

The righteous cry out, and the LORD hears,
and rescues them from all their troubles.
The LORD is near the brokenhearted;
he saves those crushed in spirit.
  Psalm 34:17–18

———

Though the fig tree does not bud and there is no
fruit on the vines, though the olive crop fails
and the fields produce no food, though the flocks
disappear from the pen and there are no herds in
the stalls, yet I will celebrate in the LORD; I will
rejoice in the God of my salvation!
  Habakkuk 3:17–18

Why, my soul, are you so dejected?
Why are you in such turmoil?
Put your hope in God, for I will still praise him,
my Savior and my God.
  Psalm 42:5

———

So you also have sorrow now. But I will see you
again. Your hearts will rejoice, and no one will take
away your joy from you.
  John 16:22

Father, I am in pain. I've lost someone dear to me during this time, and I feel that the grief is overwhelming. Lord, I know that if I stay like this, it will not help anyone. Allow me to take the grief over losing this person and turn it into joy. Allow me to remember the joy that comes from knowing and loving this person and spread that joy to others. Amen

We've all heard that laughter is the best medicine. When people struggle with illness, it seems that there is no laughter in sight, and yet, cancer research centers have used techniques like *laughter therapy* to promote a sense of health and well-being. Obviously, this is not the only form of medicine, but it certainly says something about laughter. A little bit of happiness can go a long way on the road to recovery. Take note of the things that God uses to bring joy, and focus on them. You may be surprised at the kind of good it can do for your soul.

Therefore my heart is glad
and my whole being rejoices;
my body also rests securely.
    Psalm 16:9

———

Take delight in the Lord,
and he will give you your heart's desires.
    Psalm 37:4

———

A joyful heart makes a face cheerful,
but a sad heart produces a broken spirit.
    Proverbs 15:13

I know that there is nothing better for them than to rejoice and enjoy the good life.

    Ecclesiastes 3:12

———

Rejoice in the Lord always. I will say it again: Rejoice!

    Philippians 4:4

Heavenly Father, I know that there are so many negative things that I've chosen to focus on. I know that I've allowed myself to be consumed by the negativity in my life. Allow me to focus on the things that bring happiness. Allow me to spread that happiness to others. Remind me, Lord, that this happiness comes from You. Amen

Health holds a patient's entire focus during treatment. During chemotherapy, patients have had close calls simply by catching the common cold. It's a terrifying time simply because a patient can walk into a world where nothing seemed to bother them, and now a sneeze can put their health in jeopardy. Remember that even though you may be weakened, God has blessed you to keep you moving through this weakened time. Praise God for the health that you have and keep moving forward with Him.

My flesh and my heart may fail,
but God is the strength of my heart,
my portion forever.
    Psalm 73:26

———

He heals the brokenhearted
and bandages their wounds.
    Psalm 147:3

———

*Don't be wise in your own eyes; fear the L*ORD *and*
turn away from evil. This will be healing for your
body and strengthening for your bones.
    Proverbs 3:7–8

Don't you know that your body is a temple of the Holy Spirit who is in you, whom you have from God? You are not your own, for you were bought at a price. So glorify God with your body.

1 Corinthians 6:19–20

———

So, whether you eat or drink, or whatever you do, do everything for the glory of God.

1 Corinthians 10:31

Father, thank You for my health. Thank You for giving me the ability to regain the health that I've lost. Lord, continue to be with me during this time. I know that I am weak right now, work through me to make me stronger, to make me healthier. Remind me that it is the health You've given me that has made me able to take on the obstacles that are before me now. Amen

Cancer requires honesty. It is not so much with others as much as it is with yourself. It's hard to admit to ourselves when something is wrong, especially when that something affects us on the level that cancer does. Honesty is hard. The truth has been called many things: hard, sad, ugly. It has rarely ever been referred to as anything positive. The first step to recovery is to admit that there is a problem. It takes bravery to be honest with ourselves, but we can't continue to live in denial. Take hold of Christ and move forward in truth.

Who is someone who desires life,
loving a long life to enjoy what is good?
Keep your tongue from evil
and your lips from deceitful speech.
Turn away from evil and do what is good;
seek peace and pursue it.
   Psalm 34:12–14

———

Better a poor person who lives with integrity
than someone who has deceitful lips and is a fool.
   Proverbs 19:1

———

"But let your 'yes' mean 'yes,' and your 'no' mean
'no.' Anything more than this is from the evil one."
   Matthew 5:37

Indeed, we are giving careful thought to do what is right, not only before the Lord but also before people.

    2 Corinthians 8:21

———

Do not lie to one another, since you have put off the old self with its practices.

    Colossians 3:9

Lord, I know that I have not been honest with others and myself. I know that this has put a wedge between myself and others . . . it has put a wedge between You and me. Father, I know that if I'm going to be able to move forward in life, I have to do it with honesty and with You. Lord, allow me to put down the lies in my life. Remind me of the importance and freedom that comes with honesty. Amen

Whenever the diagnosis is given, it almost always seems like all hope is lost. Doctors are very much aware of this. How do they handle it? They immediately start discussing treatment. This is often because of the fact that action must be taken quickly but also because they are working to provide the patient with a sense of hope. All of us need to feel that there is something to look forward to in times of despair. In hopeless situations, turn to God and He will provide a hope that never fails.

But those who trust in the LORD
will renew their strength;
they will soar on wings like eagles;
they will run and not become weary,
they will walk and not faint.
    Isaiah 40:31

———

I wait for the LORD; I wait
and put my hope in his word.
    Psalm 130:5

———

Now may the God of hope fill you with all joy and
peace as you believe so that you may overflow with
hope by the power of the Holy Spirit.
    Romans 15:13

We have also obtained access through him by faith into this grace in which we stand, and we rejoice in the hope of the glory of God. And not only that, but we also rejoice in our afflictions, because we know that affliction produces endurance, endurance produces proven character, and proven character produces hope.

    Romans 5:2–4

———

Let us run with endurance the race that lies before us, keeping our eyes on Jesus, the source and perfecter of our faith. For the joy that lay before him, he endured the cross, despising the shame, and sat down at the right hand of the throne of God. For consider him who endured such hostility from sinners against himself, so that you won't grow weary and give up.

    Hebrews 12:1–3

Father, I feel like there is no hope. I feel like no matter what I do I can't find success, and I know that is the problem. I can't do it on my own. Lord, be with me as I go through the hard times in life. Allow me to have a focus on You and the hope You provide. Amen

Patients often refer to their time in treatment as some of the loneliest times of their lives. You are often surrounded by people during your treatment, but there is still that element of loneliness. Even though their family may be with them, it is their path that they have to walk, and none of their loved ones can walk it with them. One of the things people point to during this time is their reliance upon those that have either walked this path before or are currently walking with them. Some patients even discuss the importance of chemotherapy in a room with others having theirs because it shows they are not alone. Know that people have walked this path and are walking it now with you, and with God you will never be alone.

"My presence will go with you, and I will give you rest."

   Exodus 33:14

———

The LORD *is the one who will go before you. He will be with you; he will not leave you or abandon you. Do not be afraid or discouraged.*

   Deuteronomy 31:8

———

God provides homes for those who are deserted.
He leads out the prisoners to prosperity,
but the rebellious live in a scorched land.

   Psalm 68:6

He heals the brokenhearted
and bandages their wounds.
    Psalm 147:3

———

Blessed be the God and Father of our Lord Jesus
Christ, the Father of mercies and the God of all
comfort. He comforts us in all our affliction, so that
we may be able to comfort those who are in any
kind of affliction, through the comfort we ourselves
receive from God.
    2 Corinthians 1:3–4

Heavenly Father, I feel so alone during this time. I know that there are others around me, but I feel like I am the only one dealing with the obstacles in my life. Lord, place people in my life that have been down the path that I am on. Place people in my life that are currently on the path that I am on. Allow me to recognize the people You have placed and continue to place in my life during this time; and remind me to respond with thankfulness. Amen

After treatment, and there are no signs of cancer, you enter a time of remission. Some patients will tell you that this is almost as mentally taxing as getting treatment because you have to be without any signs or symptoms of cancer for five years before a doctor will declare you cured. Once that time happens, however, there is an overwhelming peace that brings some patients to tears. God is the same, He provides a peace in knowing Him and that He sent His Son to die for us so that we may live forever with Him.

You will keep the mind that is dependent on you in perfect peace, for it is trusting in you.

    Isaiah 26:3

———

For I am persuaded that neither death nor life, nor angels nor rulers, nor things present nor things to come, nor powers, nor height nor depth, nor any other created thing will be able to separate us from the love of God that is in Christ Jesus our Lord.

    Romans 8:38–39

"Peace I leave with you. My peace I give to you. I do not give to you as the world gives. Don't let your heart be troubled or fearful."

    John 14:27

———

And the peace of God, which surpasses all understanding, will guard your hearts and minds in Christ Jesus. Finally brothers and sisters, whatever is true, whatever is honorable, whatever is just, whatever is pure, whatever is lovely, whatever is commendable—if there is any moral excellence and if there is anything praiseworthy—dwell on these things.

    Philippians 4:7–8

Lord, thank You for the times of peace that You have given during the times of turmoil. Allow me to continue to find those times of peace when I feel like the world is everything but peaceful. Father, allow me to put my rest in You so that I may find the peace beyond all understanding. Amen

There are normally two different kinds of patients during this process. There are those that dive into their faith, and there are those that lean on their own willpower. There are definitely some that have made it through the process on their own willpower, but the ones that have taken the time to take root in Christ and pray constantly are the ones that are able to take on the obstacles of this time and move forward with Him.

"Whenever you pray, you must not be like the hypocrites, because they love to pray standing in the synagogues and on the street corners to be seen by people. . . . But when you pray, go into your private room, shut your door, and pray to your Father who is in secret. And your Father who sees in secret will reward you. When you pray, don't babble like the Gentiles, since they imagine they'll be heard for their many words. Don't be like them, because your Father knows the things you need before you ask him.

"Therefore, you should pray like this: Our Father in heaven, your name be honored as holy. Your kingdom come. Your will be done on earth as it is in heaven. Give us today our daily bread. And forgive us our debts, as we also have forgiven our debtors. . . .

"For if you forgive others their offenses, your heavenly Father will forgive you as well. But if you don't forgive others, your Father will not forgive your offenses."

Matthew 6:5–14

*"If you remain in me and my words remain in you,
ask whatever you want and it will be done for you."*
　John 15:7

―――――

*In the same way the Spirit also helps us in our
weakness, because we do not know what to pray for
as we should, but the Spirit himself intercedes for
us with unspoken groanings.*
　Romans 8:26

―――――

*Don't worry about anything, but in everything,
through prayer and petition with thanksgiving,
present your requests to God.*
　Philippians 4:6

Lord God, There are so many things in this world that I feel like I have to accomplish. I know that I cannot do it on my own. I know that I cannot do anything during this time on my own. Allow me to not lean on my own strength and instead lean on Yours. Remind me to start my day in prayer and continue in prayer throughout the day. Remind me to pray constantly and never cease. Amen

One of the things we seek from a storm is shelter. There is not a storm quite like cancer. It is a storm most people are unequipped to handle. It is for this reason that St. Jude offers housing for families. There are so many stressors parents have to worry about when their child is dealing with cancer, and it's because of this that St. Jude works to protect families from dealing with the stress of finding lodging. When we are dealing with the storms of life, look to God, and He will protect you from what you cannot handle.

Protect me as the pupil of your eye;
hide me in the shadow of your wings.
  Psalm 17:8

———

The angel of the Lord encamps
around those who fear him, and rescues them.
  Psalm 34:7

———

The mountains surround Jerusalem
and the Lord surrounds his people,
both now and forever.
  Psalm 125:2

The name of the L<small>ORD</small> *is a strong tower;*
the righteous run to it and are protected.
    Proverbs 18:10

———

But the Lord is faithful; he will strengthen and
guard you from the evil one.
    2 Thessalonians 3:3

Heavenly Father, I feel attacked by all of the different obstacles of this season in life. I am weak and weary, and not strong enough to protect myself in this time. Lord, I know that it is only You that gives the protection that I need. Allow me to seek out that protection, Lord. Allow me to seek You as my refuge from the storms of this season and the seasons to come. Amen

One of the most common side effects in cancer treatment is fatigue. There is a weakness that comes over the body that often leaves some patients bedridden on certain days. There are some survivor stories that speak of those that got out of bed and stood, no matter what, each day. Many doctors commend these patients for their mental fortitude and spirit for being able to stand strong in a weakened state, but we know where that strength comes from. In times of turmoil, lean on God and stand with strength from Him.

My flesh and my heart may fail,
but God is the strength of my heart,
my portion forever.
  Psalm 73:26

———

But he said to me, "My grace is sufficient for you,
for my power is perfected in weakness." Therefore,
I will most gladly boast all the more about my
weaknesses, so that Christ's power may reside
in me. So I take pleasure in weaknesses, insults,
hardships, persecutions, and in difficulties, for
the sake of Christ. For when I am weak, then I am
strong.
  2 Corinthians 12:9–10

If I say, "My foot is slipping,"
your faithful love will support me, Lord.
    Psalm 94:18

———

Consider it a great joy, my brothers and sisters,
whenever you experience various trials, because
you know that the testing of your faith produces
endurance.
    James 1:2–3

Lord, I am weak. I don't have enough strength to make it on my own. I know that it is in You that I find my strength. Allow me to stand each day through the weakness and take hold of You with Your power and Your strength. Amen

A father looked at his daughter's hospital bills and began to feel stress come over him. He felt that the mountain of debt that they had incurred over the months was insurmountable. It was then that his wife took his hand and pointed to their daughter sleeping on the couch. He realized that all that stress was worth seeing his daughter sleep on something other than a hospital bed. Stress is a part of life, but it's more so about what we look to in order to get past that stress. For the father, seeing his daughter in peace was worth that stress. Look to God, let go of the stress, and give it to Him and receive peace.

Cast your burden on the L*ord,*
and he will sustain you;
he will never allow the righteous to be shaken.
    Psalm 55:22

———

Commit your activities to the L*ord,*
and your plans will be established.
    Proverbs 16:3

———

For I am the L*ord your God, who holds your right*
hand, who says to you, "Do not fear, I will help
you."
    Isaiah 41:13

"Come to me, all of you who are weary and burdened, and I will give you rest. Take up my yoke and learn from me, because I am lowly and humble in heart, and you will find rest for your souls. For my yoke is easy and my burden is light."

   Matthew 11:28–30

———

I am able to do all things through him who strengthens me.

   Philippians 4:13

Lord, I know that there are things that I cannot control. I have allowed the stress of these things to gain control over me. Father, I know that if I allow these things to stay, then I will never be able to move past them. Allow me to give this stress to You, Lord. I give this burden to You and pray You return it with peace instead. Amen

A young man had a difficult time trusting his doctor during therapy. He felt that every month he was getting weaker and weaker. He was frustrated and started accusing his doctor of not knowing what he was doing. The doctor patiently waited for the young man to finish his rant until he pulled up a fraction on his phone. The number was 567 out of 611. The doctor said, "This is the number of patients that I have treated over my twenty-seven years. Of the 611, there are 567 of those patients that are still alive. Over 90 percent of my patients are still here because they trusted me. I've treated people in worse condition than you and they still made it through because they trusted that I knew what I was doing." We act so similarly to God sometimes. We need to remember that He has been here since the beginning and that He knows us. Because of that, alone, we can put our trust in Him.

The person who trusts in the LORD, whose confidence indeed is the LORD, is blessed. He will be like a tree planted by water: it sends its roots out toward a stream, it doesn't fear when heat comes, and its foliage remains green. It will not worry in a year of drought or cease producing fruit.

    Jeremiah 17:7

———

And my God will supply all your needs according to his riches in glory in Christ Jesus.

    Philippians 4:19

———

This is the confidence we have before him: If we ask anything according to his will, he hears us.

    1 John 5:14

*Wait for the L*ORD*;*
be strong, and let your heart be courageous.
*Wait for the L*ORD*.*
  Psalm 27:14

————

"I will be with you when you pass through the
waters, and when you pass through the rivers, they
will not overwhelm you. You will not be scorched
when you walk through the fire, and the flame will
not burn you."
  Isaiah 43:2

Heavenly Father, I know that I have not trusted You. I know that I have put my trust in myself and that I should have put it in You. Lord, remind me to trust in You. Remind me to look to You each day and seek You so that I may place that trust in You. Amen

When that diagnosis is given, you become brutally aware of the fact that you are now part of a statistic. You start to worry which you'll fall in. Will you be a survivor or someone that lost the battle? The worst part about all of this is that this constant worry is something that will keep you from discovering hope. People that plant roots in worry will never grow in hope. Doctors will often point to the power of belief in the healing process. If you get tangled up in worry, the healing process seems like an impossibility. Give your worry to God and pray and believe in His healing.

"*Therefore I tell you: Don't worry about your life, what you will eat or what you will drink; or about your body, what you will wear. Isn't life more than food and the body more than clothing? Consider the birds of the sky: They don't sow or reap or gather into barns, yet your heavenly Father feeds them. Aren't you worth more than they? Can any of you add one moment to his life-span by worrying?*"

Matthew 6:25–27

———

The Lord answered her, "Martha, Martha, you are worried and upset about many things, but one thing is necessary. Mary has made the right choice, and it will not be taken away from her."

Luke 10:41–42

We know that all things work together for the good of those who love God, who are called according to his purpose.

    Romans 8:28

———

Don't worry about anything, but in everything, through prayer and petition with thanksgiving, present your requests to God. And the peace of God, which surpasses all understanding, will guard your hearts and minds in Christ Jesus.

    Philippians 4:6–7

Father, I am worried. I don't know what the future will hold and I have an uneasiness about the things in my life. Lord, allow me to give that worry to You. Allow me to find rest and guidance by living a rooted life with You. Amen

VERSE INDEX